A Doula's Guide to Nutrition

By Jemmais Keval-Baxter
The Ho'oponopono Doula™

Published by Matrilineal Ink

Published by Matrilineal Ink

Matrilineal Ink

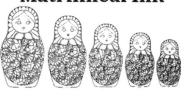

www.matrilineal.cl

Published by: Matrilineal Ink™
www.matrilineal.cl
ISBN: 978-1-9998071-4-6

A Doula's Guide
to
Nutrition

By Jemmais Keval-Baxter
The Ho'oponopono Doula™

Published by Matrilineal Ink

Published by Matrilineal Ink

Matrilineal Ink

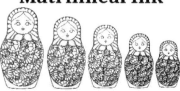

www.matrilineal.cl

Table of Contents

Introduction

Susan Weed defines excellent nutrition as "pure water, controlled breath, abundant light, loving and respectful relationships, beauty and harmony in daily life, positive, joyous thought, and vital foodstuffs."

Nutrition is everything that we put into our bodies, everything we consume, absorb through our skin and expose ourselves to through breathing.

Nutrition is of vital importance in defining our bodies, our minds, our emotions and our connection with spirit.

Optimal nutrition is the basis of all our capacities here on earth. When we are functioning at the cleanest, purest level, where our bodies are provided with all their nutritional needs, and we can protect ourselves from unnecessary toxins, then we are capable of healthy thoughts, healthy actions, healthy levels of energy, and healthy fertility. We are also able to provide the best possible environment from which to seed and grow our children.

The world is currently suffering a crisis of pollution, chemicals that are harmful to us and all other lifeforms within the various ecosystems of Earth have been released into the environment, and we do not know how long it will take for them to dissipate or be removed. The reality of the situation is that our bodies are now struggling to cope with toxins and chemicals that were never part of our ancestor's environment and that our bodies were never designed to deal with. The fact that human beings continue to populate the earth in such phenomenal numbers is a testament to the extraordinary resilience and adaptability of the human body.

Thanks to our bodies, we are able to live, and breathe, and experience light, touch, sound, taste and smell. Thanks to our bodies we have survived this long. Thanks to our bodies we are capable of reading this book. Thanks to our bodies we are capable of the most extraordinary miracle, the miracle of reproduction.

Gratitude

Gratitude is an extraordinary emotion, and like all emotions, it can change the frequency at which our bodies vibrate. Gratitude is a positive, healing and transformative emotion; it is a state of being that we as cultures and individuals need to cultivate and practice.

Take a moment out from the usual list of complaints and dissatisfactions that we have been socially programmed to focus on, and try feeling gratitude, for the overwhelmingly generous gift of life, and the body we are given to explore it with.

Thank you for all the capabilities of my body. Thank you for all that it has helped me to achieve, experience, and enjoy. Thank you for all that my body's challenges have contributed to my character, spirit, life path, purpose, empathy, understanding, and appreciation.

My body has been in constant, devoted service to me, since the moment it awakened to my soul. Thank you. I love you.

Over the last 50 years, quantum physics has demonstrated that the capacities of individual quarks, photons, electrons and the building blocks of atoms that make up our bodies and the physical world that we interact with daily, are unlimited, and they also respond to focus, will, attention and observation. This means that the way we perceive matter, effects matter, and the "natural laws" that govern our world. The nature of matter responds to perception.

Thanks to quantum physics, all scientist are mystics. If one quark can borrow energy to create itself from nothing, then miracles are possible.

Most religions, cultures, and societies, from Native American cultures to Christianity, Hinduism, Buddhism, Muslim and Judaic faiths and many others all incorporate blessings. Blessings of food and water. Our gratitude and appreciation for the gift of nature and divinity that sustain us, and our lives are blessings upon our lives and ourselves.

Taking time out and allowing yourself to intentionally feel good-feels good, it doesn't matter why. It feels good to feel good, and when we are grateful for all of the positive gifts that we have in our lives, then we are reminded of their value and can be content and satisfied, rather than anxious about acquiring or achieving more. When we integrate this gratitude and appreciation into our lives daily, choosing to focus on the positive and to feel good about ourselves, then the healing effects would speak for themselves and miracles manifest bringing us joy, peace, and fulfillment.

Attitude is key to everything. It is the key to mental health, physical survival, success, satisfaction, and fulfillment. Try it. Deicide to be happy.

Now that we are grateful for our bodies, and we are learning to be grateful for the foods and beverages that provide them with strength, renovation, building materials, and pleasures, we need to consider what kind of things we are putting into our bodies.

Nature's Gifts

Long ago, man lived from the gifts of nature, the fruits, nuts, leaves, seeds and other plant materials created by vegetation through photosynthesis. This fascinating process which combines sunlight, rainwater, and soil into life, food, and every ingredient that sustains our bodies and the bodies of all life forms, from birds and insects to reptiles, fish, and mammals.

From light to matter. **From the sunshine, we are made.**

"Know the ways of the ones who take care of you, so that you can take care of them. Introduce yourself, be accountable as the one who comes asking for life. Ask permission before taking. Abide by the answer. Never take

the first never take the last take only what you need to take only that which is given. Never take more than half, leave some for others, harvest in a way that minimizes harm. Use it respectfully. Never waste what you have taken. Share. Give thanks for what you have been given. Give a gift, in reciprocity for what you have taken. Sustain the ones who sustain you, and the earth will last forever...The deer, the sturgeon, the berries and the leeks say "if you follow these rules, we will continue to give our lives so that you may live" 1.

Within many indigenous cultural codes of ethics, we could not take from a plant or creature more than it was willing to give. We could not force the plant to produce more strawberries than it chose to, nor could we demand that nuts grow out of season, so we lived, gratefully from the gifts we were offered. The desire for strawberries demanded we wait for a full circle, a full year before they would be ready to harvest again made us even more appreciative of the flavors of our favorite foods.

As Robin Wall-Kimmerman writes in her wonderful and highly recommended book, Braiding Sweetgrass, regarding nut and trees, *"How generously they shower us with food, literally giving themselves so that we can live. But in the giving, their lives are also ensured. Our taking returns benefit to them in the circle of life making life, the chain of reciprocity. Living by the precepts of the Honourable harvest-to take only what is given, to give, to use it well, to be grateful for the gift and to reciprocate the gift."*1.

Ancient Diets

Humans have spread to nearly every corner of the world, and by necessity have adapted their eating habits, clothing styles, architecture, art and culture to the ecosystems, and the climates in which they found themselves. The reason these extraordinary distinctions between cultures have developed is due to the influence of the ecosystems in which they found themselves living. The raw building materials, cloth animal hides and edible and medicinal ingredients available to them in different locations, as well as the cycling (or not) of weather patterns and other natural phenomenon, are the foundation upon which many cultural traditions are based.

Over thousands of years, the bodies of people in isolated regions adapted to the foods that they were able to obtain to sustain themselves. This adaptability is why it is vital to consider your genetic heritage when choosing your diet. Eating the foods to which one's ancestors became accustomed is particularly crucial to our health. For example, an Inuit woman's body, adapted through generations to a sea mammal diet, with large quantities of natural fats, fish, some rare greens, and berries. She is more likely to be healthy, maintain healthy body weight, and healthy fertility, through a similar diet, than if she chooses (or is pressured through economic influences) to consume grain-based foods, such as bread, rice, pasta, and pizza.

Likewise, many people from East Asia, where a varied diet is often a well-balanced combination of fresh vegetables, meats, seafood, rice, and legumes, are more likely to be lactose intolerant since milk products have not been a regular part of their ancestor's diet.

However, for centuries, since Europe's own internal conflicts, the imperialism of Rome, slavery, religious missions and the colonization of new continents, territories, and cultures, races have mingled, and most people will find themselves of a rather varied decent. If you do come from an indigenous culture, then I encourage you to seek out a diet as closely related to your environment and your ancestor's traditional foods as possible. (By this, I mean genuinely traditional food, not necessarily adaptation foods, such as fried bread, which became traditional only after the colonization, and expulsion of native peoples from their home territories by invaders. This invasion limited the natural freedom of hunting, gathering and cultivating food, to those enforced upon them by meager and nutritionally inferior government rations.)

For the rest of us, the following guidelines are an excellent place to start.

Diets

Now before I go on, I do realize that there are a number of popular diets in the mainstream at the moment, the majority of these are designed for weight loss.... this is not what we are interested in in this book. For optimal fertility, pregnancy, childbirth, and lactation it is not advisable to pursue weight loss, as it can be very damaging to one's health and the health of the baby. Health risks associated with maternal diet can be far-reaching, affecting women's bodies after menopause, and affecting the lifelong health of a child. Sticking to a healthy diet during this period will naturally encourage our bodies to reach and sustain their optimal weight and nutrition and provide the optimal nutrition for our child.

Some of the most popular lifestyle diets are Vegetarianism, Vegan-ism, the Paleo diet, the Macrobiotic diet, the Ayurvedic diet and the Taoist diet.

Vegetarian

Vegetarianism includes the consumption of all fruits, vegetables, grains, legumes, dairy products, eggs, everything, excluding meat. That means that with this diet the intake of red meats, pork, chicken, fish, sea mammals, and wild game is prohibited. The idea is that no sentient life is sacrificed in order to feed the human individual. In many parts of the world, religious dictates have created entire cultures and nations that have sustained themselves for generations and generations on a vegetarian diet. Hindus, for example, are by religion, vegetarian, as are traditional Buddhists. They clearly demonstrate that the vegetarian diet is viable for human life.

The Ayurvedic diet, which is the vegetarian based diet of the Hindus is a system of healing and optimal health in and of itself, recommending specific ingredients, including foods, herbs, and spices, depending upon the individual characteristics of the person. There are three main Doshas or physical body types that lay the foundation for the dietary recommendations of the individual. The main Doshas are Vata, Pitta, and Kapha.

In addition to modifying the diet to those foods considered appropriate for keeping the balance of each individual, Ayurvedic practitioners advise that food should never be consumed when the consumer is feeling anxious, nervous, angry, worried or afraid. As with many holistic systems of healing, the Ayurvedic paradigm understands that emotional vibrations can influence the quality of the food that we ingest, and how it is absorbed into our bodies. It also recommends that we sit down to eat and concentrate on food when you are eating it, not reading, watching TV, driving or conversing at the same time. This is good advice for everyone, and especially those who often find themselves mindlessly snacking while doing something else, and then feeling as if they haven't eaten yet because they did not sit down to a meal. For those with an almost compulsive (OCD) desire to snack continuously while performing other tasks (or smoke...anything that involves putting things in one's mouth), it can be useful to have pure water available in a bottle, or a cup of hot unsweetened herbal tea, and consciously determine to take sips throughout your activity as an alternative to eating food, etc.

Thirst is so often misinterpreted by the body as hunger, that meeting our needs for hydration can alleviate our desire to eat in excess. When the action of eating or snacking is compulsive, due to repeatedly reinforcing this bad habit, or as a coping mechanism for anxiety, it is not the pleasure of the taste of food or beverages for which we are trying to indulge, but rather the subconscious compulsion which we choose to honor by providing a health-conscious alternative in the form of pure water.

There is a great emphasis in the Hindu vegetarian diet upon dairy products, yogurt, cream, milk, ghee (which is the refined fat from butter and may be more suitable for people with sensitivities to dairy proteins as these are removed). These products offer benefits such DHA, Vitamin A, D, K_2 and other nutrients of which ghee is a natural source, etc. The cow is a sacred animal in this culture, thanks to its endless, life-sustaining generosity, the cow represents the eternal Mother that nourishes us throughout our lives with the bountiful milk of her breast.

Ayurvedic medicine also highly praises the warming and healing nutritive powers of raw honey. However, cooked honey, or honey heated above 116ºF (which is the cut-off point before many of the vitamins, nutrients, and enzymes are destroyed), is claimed to be toxic to the body. This means no baking with honey as a substitute for sugar (instead choose maple syrup, rice syrup or other heat stable natural sugars, or even molasses), nor adding honey to boiling tea. Scientific research conducted on honey bees demonstrated that in hives where honey was extracted, heated (pasteurized) and then fed back to the bees they all died.

Dr. Weston Price emphasised the nutritional benefits of *"the deep yellow spring and fall butter from cows eating rapidly growing green grass"* as a source of vitamin A, D, E, and K_2 *"The foods that allow people of every race and every climate to be healthy are nutrient-dense natural foods— meat with its fat and especially organ meats, whole unprocessed milk products from grass-fed animals, fish, shellfish, insects, whole grains, tubers, vegetables and fruit— not newfangled concoctions made with white sugar, refined flour, processed milk and rancid, chemically altered vegetable oils—not puddings, fruit juice, sugar water and condensed milk...The diets of healthy native groups contained at least ten times more vitamin A and vitamin D than the diet of modernized peoples!"* [2.]

Dr. Price also observed that *"among traditional populations, grains, legumes, and tubers were prepared in ways that increased vitamin content and made minerals more available— soaking, fermenting, sprouting and sour leavening."* [2.]

Meat

In parts of the world where people remain dependent upon agriculture and the foods and products that they are able to produce themselves within their communities or on their own smallholding, it is usual to find a predominantly vegetarian diet, with meat being served at brief intervals throughout the year. This makes a great deal of sense for those who have an excess of only two or three male animals per year, for example, too many cockerels born means that you have roast chicken on the table. Optimally you only need one male with around 10-12 females or two males for up to 35 females, in order to continue to produce fertile eggs year-round, more than one male together will fight for mating rights.

This same rule applies to many domesticated animals, such as cows, who are naturally encouraged to produce babies on a yearly basis, to sustain their milk production. Female babies will likely be raised to produce milk and increase the herd, or sold, whereas, excess males are likely to be used for food. Sheep, are likewise raised, as are many others. Exceptions are made, some male cows are castrated to create oxen, which were traditionally used for manual labor such as tilling the soil or pulling a cart. Horses are also trained this way with the majority of male horses being castrated, and only a few bulls and stallions allowed to keep their seed for stud services, thus, ensuring future generations. Males, generally require a lot more effort to maintain, and therefore, fees for stud services are relatively high, to offset the investment.

Another critical aspect to consider is that native people, as well as those raising free-range animals themselves, had very high respect for life, they recognized the sacrifice that the animal made in order to sustain the human family, and they honored the animal and its sacrifice by wasting nothing.

This meant these people were much more likely to consume organ meats (with their higher vitamin and mineral content) than modern carnivores who can purchase their meat from a butcher and consume mostly muscle meat. Where the life of the animal sacrificed to sustain the life of the people is honored, many consider the animals to be their brethren, flesh of their flesh. Kin.

In the wild, many herd animals, reindeer, caribou, and others such as lions and some whales, tend to organize themselves into large family groups, or prides (in the case of lions), where many females and their offspring live together communally, with only one wild stallion, two male lions (usually brothers), or a few male caribou for herd numbers that can reach the hundreds, even thousands of females during migration.

These groups are the fertile groups that produce future generations. Females stay together in communities, and males fight over the right to be accepted by them as the strongest, best protector, who will father their offspring, watch over them, and protect them from harm, as they independently forage or hunt for food.

The excess males are booted out of the group and often roam together in groups for company and protection, rarely fighting amongst themselves unless in the presence of females, to which they feel obliged to show off for and compete over. Males on their own are easier targets for predators and are very unlikely to have a chance at mating and propagating their genes unless they take over another male's pride or herd. It is interesting to observe. Females will often decide collectively to reject males. Even when they have bested the previous top-ranked male and females refuse to include them in their community, despite their individual strength; a single male is no match for the collective power of the females.

However, this is not the rule for all animals. Birds for example often mate and raise eggs and young in pairs, though rarely staying faithful to a pairing beyond each year, having to find and win over a new mate each season. Some parrots, of course, are known to mate for life, often committing suicide when their lover dies.

Egg-laying fish and reptiles rarely interact for longer than the mating dance. Wolves are relatively distinct, in that their social structure is hierarchical and includes many males and females, often related. Only the alpha female has the right to reproduce, and it is her choice as to mate with which male. More often than not, she will choose the alpha male, as he is demonstrated to be of high quality (otherwise he wouldn't be a leader). The entire pack raises the young as their own, and thus, the number of wolves in the pack is sustainable since only one female will produce one litter at each time.

Prey animals that herd naturally produce more offspring since many are lost to predators, and in order to sustain their numbers rather than being exterminated, they reproduce quickly. This process is why herd animals have been humans first choice for domestication and productivity.

Another reason that many animals domesticated for food are herbivores is that environmental toxins and pollutants can accumulate as they move up the food chain. When a plant grows, it absorbs a certain amount of toxicity from its environment, from contaminants in the water, air, and soil, the more pollutants it is exposed to the more it will absorb. When an insect, bird or other animal consumes these plants they absorb those toxins into their body, and they accumulate, concentrating in the animals flesh the more they consume. Most of the meat that is eaten in the western world is of purely herbivorous animals. When a carnivore eats the meat of that herbivore, it will absorb the contaminants in that flesh, and because carnivores eat many animals, they absorb the contaminants from all the animals and plants they themselves consumed concentrating them further. Therefore carnivores have higher levels of contaminants and toxins in their bodies than herbivores. This is also true for fish as it is for other carnivorous animals, (pigs and goats are omnivores like dogs, and are known to eat anything and everything including feces, which is why any culture consider them unclean and unfit to consume).

Toxins in Our Fat

Thanks to decades worth of irresponsible dumping of toxic waste into the sea, including toxic metals, radioactive and medical waste, raw sewage and any number of chemical run-offs from factories, the world's oceans have been severely contaminated and overloaded.

Predatory fish, at the top of the food chain, such as shark and tuna, swordfish (Merlin) and mackerel accumulate a higher concentration of mercury and other toxic metals because they consume other fish and absorb the toxins from their bodies. Tony Robbins was apparently gravely ill after suffering mercury poisoning which he attributes to the high quantities of swordfish and other predator fish in his diet. He has specifically designed a simple diet for himself based upon the rotation of certain vegetables, grains, and seafood, to maintain optimal health. He was devastated to find out that he had been unwittingly poisoning himself with high doses of mercury due to the contamination of the ocean and all seafood when he had been so self-disciplined in his nutritional choices.

Toxins that the body are unable to deal with immediately, such as toxic metals, herbicides, and other environmental pollutants are often stored in body fat. When our body has too high of a toxic load (think binging on junk-food, caffeine, alcohol on a day to day basis), then the liver is unable to process it all at once. The body responds by storing toxins in fat; the idea is to save the extra work for night-time or the next day or moment when the liver has time to dedicate itself to this extra work. Unfortunately, if we continue to overload our system with toxins the liver never has a chance to clear the backlog of toxins stored in the fat and the body is forced to produce more and more fat to store the toxins while they wait to be processed.

When someone fasts or goes on a detox program, what they are doing is merely eliminating any additional toxins, so that the liver can clear the backlog. The body always heals itself if we just provide it with the opportunity. Therefore many people experience detox reactions, feeling unwell for several days while starting the fast since the toxins previously stored in fat tissues are released and need to be processed and eliminated by the liver.

Because environmental toxins are often stored in fats, the animal fats we consume in our diets are also potential sources of these toxins. This is one of the convincing health arguments for a plant-based vegetarian or vegan diet. Consuming organic, wild harvested, or free range, pastured meat, fish and dairy products are especially important if you choose to retain these items as a part of your diet. One of the advantages of raising your own animals for food or dairy products is your ability to ensure their health by preserving their exposure to a natural diet, clean air, sunshine, and exercise.

Fatty fish such as salmon was once considered to be extremely healthy. However, controversial farming techniques that rely upon overcrowding, broad-spectrum antibiotics and feeding with food pellets, has damaged salmon's reputation with consumers as a source of healthy fats and proteins, as well as having had a detrimental impact on many natural and once diverse ecosystems. The media's recent coverage of the catastrophic impact that global salmon farming has had on the seas around Chiloe is enough to convince many socially and environmentally responsible consumers to take salmon off the menu.

The quality of meat from an animal that has been pastured on the land, eating fresh grasses and other forage, under the sun, sky and the elements is vastly different than an animal that has suffered through industrial farming methods, sacrificing their life and their quality of life for the sake of economic profit. *"Epinephrine (adrenaline) and nor-epinephrine are "stress hormones" that when released into the bloodstream will stay in the body and the effect the quality of the meat. When you eat this excited animal meat, you are ingesting those hormones and hormone-induced by-products in your body. Consuming this type of meat can cause unwanted health problems in your system."* [3.]

"The goddess never wasted her substance without recycling; Every living form served as nourishment for other forms. Every blossom fed an organic rot. Everything had its day in the sun, then gave place to others, which made use of its dying." [4.]

I advise everyone to go out and learn a variety of healthy vegetarian recipes for main dishes. The modern western diet has accustomed people to think a meal must include meat, chicken, or fish of some kind (otherwise it's not a meal). Most people, therefore, consume at least two portions of meat a day, in sandwiches, wraps, stir-fries, takeaways, roasts, bacon and egg breakfasts, etc. This is excessive, not only for our bodies' health and digestion but also in terms of the earth's resources. If we are to learn once again to live sustainably with what the earth can provide and gift to us in such a way that next year, there will be an equal (not less) bounty, then we must learn to adjust our eating patterns.

There are a large variety of vegetarian dishes available, from all over the world, that taste fantastic and are by no means lacking in meat. If you are a meat eater, try to reduce your intake of meat and fish to two servings per week or less.

That means a couple of meals per week may include meat or fish of your choice, but for the remainder of the time, you choose your meals and snack from the vegetarian options. If you are cooking at home, this may even help to reduce your food budget.

If you choose to consume meat, I advise a variety of meals using nutrient-dense organ meats, such as the liver and kidneys, as these were a significant part of our ancestors' diets (all people surviving from the land, be it hunting and gathering or agriculture, and domestication of livestock would be unwilling to waste). Liver in particular (and cod liver oil if you just are not accustomed to eating liver on a regular basis) is an abundant source of a variety of essential vitamins including vitamin A, D, B_6, B_{12}, K_2, and DHA.

"until the end of the second world war, cod liver oil served as the number one supplement for pregnant women and growing children...in order to protect themselves from infectious disease and ensure strong bones and {straight} teeth...liver was considered a sacred food in almost all traditional cultures, necessary for strength, stamina and for the production of beautiful, healthy children...Cod liver oil also provides an important omega-3 fatty acid called DHA, docosahexaenoic acid, needed for brain development." [2]

Taste

It is necessary for many of us raised in an era of processed, convenience foods, to retrain our taste-buds to listen to the actual needs of our bodies, as our bodies are always communicating with us, and it is in our best interest to learn to listen to and interpret this information well.

"The average American consumes nine pounds of additives per year, including preservatives, dyes, bleaches, emulsifiers, antioxidants, artificial and "natural" flavors, conditioners, extenders, anti-caking agents, and thickeners." 2.

Our bodies were designed to live from the gifts of nature, this may or may not have included hunting animals (likely the excess males rather than the breeding females) or not, depending upon your ideology. In the wild, certain types of foods, such as carbohydrates and sugars, that supply much of the energy for our bodies (which is why many weight loss diets exclude these foods). These are not as available, and more time consuming to produce; either from cultivated grain (we have as whole bean agriculture, rather than hunter and gatherer for a very long time and our bodies have likewise adapted to this transformation) or from the harvesting of roots and tree starch.

When a lot of effort is expended to produce the food that is acquired, then mathematically you can see that the calorific value of the food balances the calories utilized by the body, and therefore, weight is maintained. Fruits and wild honey, the sweets of nature, provide sugars at very little energy loss for harvest. Likewise, the fats from seeds and nuts and lean wild animals (breastfed babies carrying the highest levels of body fat....thus the popularity of lamb) would have been rare.

Our ancestors would not have had a regular excess of harvest from nuts and seeds, allowing them to produce liters and liters of vegetable oils for cooking throughout the year. As a result, the domestication of animals and the milking of them to produce butter, milk, yogurt, cheese, ghee, and other fat-rich foods was another revolutionary addition to the human diet.

Salt intake, other than for those regularly consuming seafood, would have been relatively rare. Salt is a sign of high mineral content in foods as many rock salts, and the salts contained within plants, are accompanied by necessary minerals that the body values highly.

In a natural diet that is dependent upon harvesting from nature, sugars and sweet tasting things, fats, and salts were the flavors that our bodies craved beyond anything else, their relative scarcity, meant that we eagerly sought them out whenever they became available to supplement our diet and replenish our reserves. Taste and desire were how our bodies communicated with us, teaching us to seek out the nutrients that we needed to thrive and prosper.

In the modern diet, food has been so profoundly and extensively manipulated that much of foods are now highly supplemented with an excess of sugar, salt, and fat. Our body still craves these things. We have not had so many generations of access that our bodies have become adapted to the abundance and changed our perceptions of taste, yet our eating habits have educated our taste buds to seek out stronger and stronger stimulants.

If you have ever eaten a piece of fruit after consuming sugar, in the form of candy, chocolate bars or jam, the fruit will taste sour rather than sweet. Our sensitivity to the sweetness of the fruit has been diminished, and so we taste the other flavors of the fruit instead, (incidentally this also occurs after cleaning your teeth as most toothpaste contains artificial sweeteners or in the case of some natural fluoride free toothpaste- stevia extracts).

The same is true of salt. When the body is accustomed to eating foods prepared without salt, a small pinch added to the food is noticeable. However, someone accustomed to salt at every meal (and salt is added even to bread, pastries and sweet things let alone to the water in which potatoes are cooked, etc.) the salt will go unnoticed, and the lack of salt will be missed, though not always automatically identified. Salt has become associated with flavor. When we are able to clean our pallet (this can take as little as a couple of weeks), then our sensitivity to flavor is heightened, and we are better able to enjoy the various and subtle flavors available in fresh, natural foods, without the need for additional stimulants.

Cleaning one's pallet is very important. The first two weeks of a new diet can be the most challenging, for example, the first two weeks without additional salt can make everything taste flavorless, or the first two weeks without a stimulant such as coffee can leave your body feeling sluggish, as it adjusts its neuron-transmitters to a new baseline. The same is true for sweets. If you cut out all sweet things, including artificial sweeteners from your diet for two weeks, then you may feel that you miss it. Entirely cutting out sugar can result in some very dramatic withdrawal symptoms. But after a period your awareness of taste and sweetness will be enhanced, and a reduced serving of half a teaspoon of honey in your herbal tea will taste rewardingly sweet.

Every child is born with a clean pallet. They are born seeking breast-milk and nothing else. After four months they may have the desire to taste or suck at other foods, these aid in teething and may indicate a desire to include iron in their diet, but it is not until six months that children should be encouraged to eat semi-solid foods. Every child will adapt his or her taste buds to the food that (s)he was exposed to during infancy, (and to a certain extent to the diet of the mother during pregnancy). No child is born craving artificially colored sweets or Coca-Cola, or crisps or any other man-made highly unnatural and health-damaging foods. So, if parents could learn to educate their children from the beginning to enjoy a healthy diet, they will continue to enjoy that diet for the rest of their lives, and be blessed with the best possible health that they can achieve. How could a loving parent wish for anything better than that?

There is a false and disgusting rumor that some children don't like eating vegetables, which is ridiculous. Vegetables constitute the primary source of nutrients for our bodies for most people in most parts of the world and are therefore naturally attractive to children exposed to them. Any attitude against eating vegetables or fruits is adopted by the child mimicking a bad example set by the people around them.

Sugar

I have seen people give "treats" of a spoonful of sugar to their children, which they consider to be a gift (not that much different than giving hard-boiled sweets, fudge, toffee, lollipops and other candy). From my perspective, knowing what I do about the physiology of the human body, its needs and physical, emotional, hormonal reactions to sugar, I see this as dangerous, a spoonful of poison. *"The metabolism of sugar uses up large amounts of vitamins, minerals, and enzymes and creates a roller-coaster of high and then low blood sugar levels. The list of conditions caused by consumption of sugar is a long one. The conditions include: diabetes, hypoglycemia, frequent infectious illness, heart disease, cancer, digestive problems, endocrine problems, infertility, skin problems, obesity, increased desire for alcohol, coffee, and tobacco, Candida overgrowth, bone loss, dental decay, hyperactivity, violent tendencies, and depression."*[2.]

If it did not taste so pleasant to those who were taught to consume it, then the damage to the teeth alone would be enough to discourage a parent from administering it to child.

If we saw a drug addict give some of their drugs to their baby, we would be outraged. The parent would naturally consider the drug a gift, since it makes them feel so good. However, we would see all of the damage (and potential lifelong struggle to resist the unnecessary cravings) done by the drug. This behavior would be child abuse. Sugar is 100 times more addictive than cocaine. And it is directly responsible and adversely linked to diseases such as diabetes, heart disease, Candida yeast infections, incapacitated immune defense, cancer, joint inflammation, dental decay, emotional disorders, eating disorders, fungal infections, hyperactivity, reduced concentration, memory and mental skills impairment, and numerous other unbalances in the system.

"Poorly digested grains and pasteurized milk create dietary opiates, excitotoxins, and cannabinoids that mimic morphine, heroin, and marijuana. Sugar produces dopamine and endorphins that mimic cocaine, morphine, opium, and heroin as sugar stimulates the production of adrenaline and norepinephrine, which mimic methamphetamine. In addition, sugar feeds yeasts that can produce ethanol and acetaldehyde, resulting in symptoms of inebriation and hangover. Artificial sweeteners such as aspartame, artificial flavors such as MSG and hydrolyzed protein, and emulsifiers such as carrageenan produce glutamate, a powerful brain stimulant that can be toxic in large amounts. When children are ingesting these foods, can we blame them for fussiness, whining, crying, crabbiness, sullenness, tantrums, insomnia and general bad behavior?" [2.]

If a child is always taught to enjoy fresh fruits and appreciate cooked vegetables, then that child will never have to struggle to counteract poor eating habits or long for "forbidden foods" that they never learned to crave.

Refined sugar strips the body of nutrients that it already has, in order for the sugar entering the system to be processed. These nutrients, if not replaced, become deficiencies, and if this is repeated the body can become malnourished.

"Refined sugar is a thief. Period. Where dairy is adding unnecessary gunk to your closets, sugar is sneaking jewel after jewel out of your treasure chest. You see, when your body is faced with sugar to digest, it provides all the missing bits and pieces taken away in the refinement of sugarcane. Add your personal store of minerals to the mix. So, it's not even that sugar is a thief. Sugar is like a bad guest that comes to your home and does a giddy little jig in the living room for about fifteen minutes, creating a great euphoria for the whole family. Suddenly the dance ends, she picks up an ax, and proceeds to smash and slash all the furniture in the house. With sugar, we lose B vitamins, calcium, phosphorus, iron, and peace of mind... If you have never kicked sugar before, you may not know the withdrawal it puts a human through depression, lethargy, intense cravings, anger, negativity, night sweats, nightmares, crying." [5.]

The nutrients available in natural food, vitamins, minerals, amino acids, etc., are the necessary building blocks for our bodies to grow (as children, or a fetus in utero), to function and repair themselves. Just like workmen, if we do not provide enough of the right materials, the body simply cannot do its job. Only so many substitutions can be made before the structure is weakened and becomes vulnerable to the attack of an opportunistic parasite, virus or bacteria seeking a hospitable environment, making our bodies ill. The deterioration from wear and tear of the body through ordinary activity, comparable to a house exposed to the elements, must be maintained or become derelict, eventually crumbling and falling down.

In nature, sugars available from fruits, and honey, and even sugar cane are not isolated, they come available in a package. Nature provides everything in context, so all of the nutrients needed to assimilate the food are included in the food (avoiding any problems with digestion). In addition, each food contains an abundance of characteristics, instrumental in hydration, energy, vitamins, minerals, taste and color vibrations, that all contribute to the optimal healthy working of the body. These are currently referred to as whole foods.

Nature is much smarter than us humans. Nature is adept at creating. Scientific history is a continuous story of man's discovery of something; isolation of a specific ingredient, or the abuse of another ingredient without harmony and balance. Then there is the discovery that one ingredient works best in combination with other ingredients that are, by coincidence, often discovered in the same place as the initially isolated ingredient, already provided by nature.

This scenario also applies to medicines, all of which have their origins in plants, herbs, and minerals, etc. Nature provides compounds because nature understands the concepts of symbiosis, cooperation, and reciprocity. Nature knows that nothing in the universe works in isolation, everything works as a team. Nature spent millions of years creating systems (universal, and microscopic) that interact sustainably, and we, as humans are slowly coming to appreciate all of her infinite wisdom. It is time that we set about restoring balance since humans have been mostly responsible for interfering with all of the perfectly choreographed cycles of life and health on this multi-species planet that is our home.

We cannot treat the earth as if it were disposable, for her existence and our own are indistinguishable, without the nurturing abundance of her gifts, how would we ever survive?

Vegetarian food is not by definition healthy, many processed foods are made meat-free, but lack the nutritive value to support optimal health, so more is required. Be careful.

Veganism

Veganism is a stricter form of vegetarianism, where all animal products, including honey, eggs, dairy products, etc. are also off-limits. Some information on the internet suggests that vegan cultures have existed in the past, including citing the possibility of a 5,000-year-old vegan Brok-pa Aryan community in the Himalayas, although, there is contention regarding these claims and many refute their strict adherence to a vegan diet. Many more cultural examples can be found in which around 90% of the people are vegan although, there is a great deal of speculation as to the verification of long-term vegan societies.

Modern methods of monoculture cultivation accompanied by mass applications of herbicides and pesticides have resulted in a depletion of nutrients in the foods that we consume and the micro-organisms that live in the soil. Many vegans cite this as the reason why today's vegan diet lacks the essential vitamin B12. Modern Vegans, as a rule, choose to supplement this vitamin to their diet. Possibly negligent hygiene may have resulted in ancient "vegans" to consume more insects and other life forms in their foods, which would not be considered appropriate by today's standards, for a variety of reasons.

The vegan diet, like the vegetarian diet, is not necessarily healthy as it can just as easily include fizzy pop and fried crisps. However, it can be healthy when approached sensibly and with balance.

Raw Veganism

Raw Vegans, as the name, suggests eating only raw foods, including fruits, vegetables, nuts, seeds, sea vegetables, fermented pickles, sprouts and other natural products that have not been heated above 116ºF. This diet is very popular, not just for weight loss (dramatic results have been reported), but also as a long-term lifestyle choice. Food quantity is not limited on this diet, only quality, where the healthiest, most natural, organic or biodynamic products are favored.

During times of illness, and even as a regular practice for health throughout the year, fasting, or reducing intake to raw foods, is very healthy, and advised in many religions. Eating raw foods preserve the natural enzymes, and arguably higher levels of nutrients such as vitamins and minerals (some of which would likely degrade during the cooking process), allowing for easier digestion. The body, once freed of the extra work of digesting heavy and problematic foods has more energy to devote to healing and rejuvenation.

Whole foods, which are predominantly the choice of raw vegans also have higher levels of fiber and hydration. Trials have demonstrated remarkable results in a number of acute and chronic conditions when individuals adhere to a strict raw food diet for a period of 30-60 days. In addition to 'feeling better,' one trial on diabetes found all of the participants reduced the severity of their condition from medicated diabetes that required daily injections of insulin to diet controlled diabetes (that is, they had no symptoms of diabetes while eating the raw food diet and required no medication).

As I mentioned the raw food diet does not limit intake, so it is possible to eat carbohydrate-rich bananas and fatty avocado pears to your heart's content, (and you should since they provide so many positive nutrients). This kind of diet is particularly suited to warm climates and summer weather, where our bodies naturally communicate to us a desire for fresher, lighter food, with higher levels of hydration. However, some people have experienced the feeling of being excessively cold on a raw food diet during the winter. Many raw food communities can be found in sunny climates such as California, Hawaii, Australia, and Thailand.

While everything available to eat on the raw food diet is of the very best nutritional value and should make up the majority of most peoples diets; as with regular veganism, there are certain essential nutrients not readily available and need to be supplemented. Some radical raw food activists argue that cows, oxen, horses and other strong mammals consume the raw food diet. People are in fact the only creatures on the planet that cook their food – this came from our expansion to less hospitable environments where it became necessary to seek out additional food and cooking to remove parasites, bacteria and other pathogens or toxins for the sake of survival. Herbivores in the wild synthesize vitamin B12 and all the other nutrients they need by themselves from sunlight and the raw food diet, with the help of gastrointestinal flora. It is proposed that given the opportunity, the human body, should be capable of the same, once the genetic information we have not used for countless generations is re-activated.

I have 100% faith in the capacities of the human body, they are potentially unlimited, so I cannot argue with the possibility that we can adapt in such a way. However, it takes extraordinary capacities of spirit to evolve to such miraculous levels of being. And unfortunately, the reality of the situation at present is that many people who have been on the raw food diet for years find that their bodies eventually run out of B_{12} reserves and that at that point, for the sake of their health they wisely choose to supplement their diet with this nutrient.

There may have been a time when gut flora was able to synthesize adequate levels of Vitamin B_{12} as it does vitamin K. However, the majority of modern people have significantly depleted the diversity of helpful bacteria in their intestines, in comparison to our ancestors who consumed a large quantity of Lacto-fermented products. They also did not use pesticides, herbicides, disinfectants, and antibiotics in the same way that we do now in our vendetta against germs.

"When we wipe out the beneficial bacteria—that are extremely vulnerable to broad-spectrum antibiotics, contraceptive pill, steroid medications prescribed on a long-term basis, and in fact, to the majority of modern drugs that are used on a repeat prescription basis—we end up with what is called gut dysbiosis (damaged gut flora)." 6.

The Weston Price Foundation states that *"vitamin K2 is found in fermented foods such as natto, sauerkraut and grass-fed animal fats— goose liver, cheese, and to a lesser extent butter, egg yolks"* [6.] This means that there are some vegan sources available, however, if you are vegan it may be necessary to supplement B12 and K2 since the amount of sauerkraut you would need to consume to support yourself through pregnancy may not be appetizing. Nutritional yeast flakes are often considered a healthy vegan source of B vitamins. Although, there is some contention regarding the propensity of this substance to feed yeast and fungus in the intestines, that could potentially contribute to the overgrowth of Candida. Candida (a wild yeast found in most people's bodies) feeds on sugar and is a blight on many a raw vegans life.

The raw food diet is stringent. For many people seeking to maintain a lifelong commitment to the diet, strategies have evolved. Some people supplement their raw vegan diet with other raw products such as raw eggs, raw honey, raw milk, yogurt, and cheese. Obviously, these are not vegan, and as they are unpasteurized, the raw products carry a higher risk of contamination such as botulism from honey, salmonella from eggs and tuberculosis from milk products. For this reason, it is imperative to seek reliable sources. The website www.realmilk.com is a valuable resource for the Western Price Foundation that has a list of raw milk suppliers in the U.S.A. Another alternative is to raise your own dairy animals or keep chickens and bees in your backyard. Raw cheeses are much easier to find as they are sold in mainstream shops. Others choose to follow a 75-85% raw vegan diet, eating cooked food for 15% of the time.

Another strategy that is often recommended for those seeking to transition into a raw food diet is to eat raw food throughout the day and have one cooked meal in the evening. This is a beneficial option for many pregnant women, especially if they feel particularly sensitive and nauseous in the mornings. Nausea during pregnancy is simply the body's form of cleansing, detoxifying and communicating its nutritional needs and the nutritional needs of the baby to you. The more that you listen to your body's advice, the easier it will be for you as you will be giving your body and your baby what they need.

Some women who have experienced substantial toxic exposure for years leading up to their pregnancy, from drug or alcohol consumption, taking the contraceptive pill or working in an environment saturated with toxins such as a hairdressing salon paint studio or gas station, will have a higher need to detoxify during pregnancy. As a result, these women may suffer more intensely with nausea or vomiting. Therefore it is often advised to take a period of one to two years to detoxify your life and your body and the life of your partner and their body when considering conscious conception before you get pregnant.

Diet and lifestyle have an extraordinary influence on fertility and many women struggling to conceive have found success after switching to a healthy diet. The motivation to conceive a child can be profoundly inspiring, and the transition to a healthy lifestyle can have a positive benefit on the lives of the parents and the child for the rest of their lives. This is often a unique lesson and blessing to come out of the situation that men and women find themselves in when facing fertility issues.

I do not advise that any woman adopt a 100%, vegetarian, vegan or raw vegan during pregnancy or lactation if they are not accustomed to it, as the adaptation can be challenging for the body and during pregnancy and breastfeeding the need to provide for the fetus and produce milk is already taxing enough. However, many women have successfully given birth and raised healthy children when adhering to their long-term vegetarian, vegan and raw vegan diets, just as many women have been fortunate enough to raise healthy children on a diet of fast food and sugary drinks (but I don't advise that for anyone's health either).

The Essenes

The Essene is a religious order that follows a strict diet based upon advice extracted from some of the ancient Dead Sea Scrolls, recovered from the Vatican archives. Translations of the specific scrolls that they consult regarding diet can be found on the internet if you search for the Gospel of the Essene. According to the translation, Jesus advised people to eat only living food, (raw food) which contained all the positive life force of nature. Essene follow a raw food diet (a little stricter than the average raw foodstuff in that they are not permitted to eat cooked food, frozen food or fermented food). They are advised to eat fruits and vegetables available to them from their own land. In season, drying fruit is acceptable, and a recipe in the Gospel of the Essene (reportedly recommended by Jesus himself) for daily bread was made from sprouted grains, which were milled, formed into flat unleavened biscuits and baked only by the heat of the sun.

Presuming that this advice was given in a hot, arid desert region, I imagine that using a dehydrator may be a possible adaptation for colder climates. According to the Gospel of the Essene, this diet of living food, should restore the body to health and keep it healthy for a long and extended period of life. Many claims that this living diet was what helped so many of Adam's descendants (mentioned in the Bible) to live lifetimes spanning hundreds of years. Sprouting seeds and grains releases a great deal of nutrients and aids in the digestion of these grass seeds that would otherwise have to be cooked.

Paleo

The Paleo diet has been gaining popularity over the last few years. The premise is food included within the diet is that it is akin to the diet of our paleolithic ancestors. The Paleo diet consists of unlimited lean meats, fruits, and non-starchy vegetables. However, the diet eliminates dairy products, processed foods, cereals, legumes, and limits starchy root vegetables such as potatoes, sweet potatoes, tapioca, yams, plantains, and taro.

"Paleo" style diets allow nuts and seeds but not grains and beans because many of our ancestors would likely have been eating nuts and seeds long before the invention of agriculture. Most nuts and some seeds do not require any processing to be edible, whereas, all grains and legumes must be soaked, fermented, and/or thoroughly cooked in order to be digestible. This is a fantastic diet for those that choose to eat meat with a dairy and gluten intolerance since it forbids all bread and grain-based baked goods, providing possible alternatives with almond flour and ground flaxseed, etc. Even if you do not intend to follow the Paleo diet, it is worth reading through some recipes they recommend as alternatives, as it may inspire you in the kitchen, open up your creativity and introduce you to new possibilities, especially when you may not have your usual ingredients on hand.

Gluten and Dairy Free

The gluten and dairy free diet have been recommended and proven therapeutically effective in children suffering from regressive-autism, (this is a kind of autism that develops in early childhood often after exposure to toxic or traumatic experiences). Many parents claim a link to the Thimerosal (mercury) content and other toxic ingredients of childhood vaccines which resulted in seemingly healthy children who were developing speech, motor control and social skills to ceasing development and actually regressing, losing speech, demonstrating aggressive behavior, inability to maintain eye contact, often developing long-term diarrhea and other signs of an inflamed digestive system, as well as many other issues.

Many parents attribute the extra sensitivity of children suffering from autism spectrum to processed foods, sugars, dairy products and gluten, and believe that this is a sign to all of us that these products should not be a part of our diet.

High levels of superfoods and other supplementation of vitamins and minerals, often missing from these children's systems (possibly through inefficient digestion due to inflammation and sensitivity of the gut) are also recommended, as well as keylation (a medical procedure to extract toxic heavy metals from the body).

A reduction of wheat products is good advice for everyone. Even if you have not been identified as having a gluten intolerance, since wheat is in so many of our foods, especially heavily processed and refined white flours, which can build up in our digestive system. I recall arts and crafts projects for children which included making makeshift "glue" out of four and water; it is the gluten in the flour that produces this sticky glue-like consistency. There is concern about a build-up of this "glue" clogging up the bowels leading to constipation, IBS, and other digestive problems.

Saiten which is often sold as an alternative meat substitute for vegetarians is made from pure gluten; some people even make their own by washing wheat-flour until all that is left is the rubbery gluten which they cook and flavor as a substitute for meat.

Gerson Therapy

Another therapeutic diet developed to help people recover from all types of health issues, from terminal illnesses to addictions, poor eyesight, eczema, and allergies is the Gerson Therapy, which emphasizes a strict vegetarian based diet and copious amounts of juice. The juicing of large quantities of fresh fruits and vegetables is reported to feed the body high doses of vitamins and minerals to offset any malnourishment (said to be an epidemic in the modern industrialized world). It is thought to promote the body's own healing capacities, in as easily digestible form as possible, and without the prohibitive excess of eating fruits and vegetables in bulk every day. It is a diet worth investigating for anyone interested in healing, either as a long-term solution to illness or for a short-term detox.

Macrobiotics

The macrobiotic diet is one of the most famously healthy lifestyle diets available. Many people who have been diagnosed with terminal illnesses such as cancer have adopted a macrobiotic diet to help cleanse their body of toxins and promote the body's natural healing capacities. There have been several success stories, and a great number of people have sustained a macrobiotic lifestyle for generations. The macrobiotic diet is very clean and is based upon the traditional diet of the Japanese working peasants.

Like most people working from the land, they had limited amounts of meat and fish, a greater variety of fresh vegetables from their gardens, seasonal fruits and the foundation of their diet consisted of carbohydrates in the form of whole grains. Most starchy root vegetables such as potatoes and yams were not available, in fact, potatoes, tomatoes, bell peppers, and aubergines, which all belong to the same plant family as the poisonous belladonna, deadly nightshade, are poisonous to the system and are to be avoided in the macrobiotic diet. Every grain and vegetable etc. is deemed to have a balance. Other foods such as brown rice are considered to be perfectly balanced in relation to people and can, therefore, be eaten daily. However other grains had various nutritional properties and needed to be rotated. As with many different healthy diets, whole foods are emphasized, and all refined and processed foods are rejected. Fruits and fruit juices are limited in this diet, however, as are most sweeteners, except for organic brown rice syrup which is recommended for use only in moderation. Modern recipes suggest a laxer interpretation of the proportions of food on the Macrobiotic diet.

This diet is considered to be a very economical one. It is suitable for situations in which people rely heavily on dried foods which can be stored long-term without refrigeration (such as camping, traveling, survival, etc., since dried grains, flours, fruits, and seeds last well, and can be purchased cheaper in bulk to last for a long time.

Macrobiotics encourage eating large amounts of sea vegetables (very healthy and rich in iodine) and to scrub rather than peel all fruits and vegetables consumed, as every part of the plant, including the skin is thought to provide nutrients. This demonstrates a respect for the balance designed by nature for each plant. It has been demonstrated by science that a lot of nutrients occur in the skins of apples and root vegetables such as sweet potatoes, swedes, parsnips, carrots, beetroot's, etc. A unique brush is available to scrub vegetables. However, it is most appropriately used with organic vegetables (not a problem when you grow your own) since higher levels of pesticides, herbicides, and chemical fertilizer residue can be found on the surface of fruits and vegetables cultivated under modern industrial farming conditions.

In macrobiotics, the spirit and energetic consistency of each ingredient is strictly identified and highly respected. It is not only necessary to consider the health benefits of each ingredient individually, but also in relation to one another in terms of taste, color, male and female energy (yin vs. yang), the time of year and the method of preparation. Balance is the essence.

Grains not only form the basis of the macrobiotic diet but are considered sacred. Each whole grain, no matter how long it is stored, contains the dormant essence of life, that when awakened has the capacity to grow and produce a new plant, even generations of plants. The energy within the grain is contained, concentrated and infinitely patient. Many report a greater sense of peace and well-being when they are on a macrobiotic diet and attribute their perception of calm and centered tranquillity to the nature of grains, which are wise, ageless and potent. There certainly seems to be a correlation between a healthy diet and healthy emotional states; mood swings are often substantially contributed to by the roller-coaster of blood sugar levels which result from a processed food heavy modern diet. Children diagnosed with ADHD respond very well to routine exercise and whole food diets such as macrobiotics.

Whole Foods

The ancient Greek philosopher Hypocrites is often quoted as being the founder of modern medicine, although, much of his knowledge was influenced by Arabic slaves, traditional midwives, and other wise herbalists. Hippocrates stated, *"Let medicine be your food and let food be your medicine."* A wonderful guiding principle for designing you and your family's eating habits.

Every whole food ingredient that we use, whether it is meat, vegetable, herb or spice, contains specific nutritional, and phytochemical (plant chemical) components. In order to be healthy and to stay healthy, we should not be waiting until we are unwell and out of balance to treat symptoms with medication (be it herbal, or pharmaceutical). Our goal should be to obtain and maintain optimal health from the beginning to avoid illness or susceptibility to disease.

To ensure that our body has all of the nutrients it needs it is recommended we consume as varied a diet as possible, including as many different whole food ingredients as possible. In Japan, it is recommended by the government that everyone eat a minimum of 30 different ingredients per day (that means 30 unique raw ingredients, not baked potato, potato chips, potato fries and hash browns; which are variations of the same ingredient)

Our ancestors are thought to have included more than 350 raw ingredients in their diet, simply due to their need to survive and the lack of over-abundance of any one type of food available. Today's diet is over saturated with an abundance of foods produced in large quantities from monoculture. Ingredients such as potatoes, corn, rice, wheat, soy, and sugar are processed and reinvented into hundreds of different products. While adding variety to our eyes and taste-buds, these products do not add nutritional variety. If we eat only the same foods repeatedly, then we will miss out on any nutrients that are unavailable in these foods, which will result in a nutrient deficiency.

It is an extraordinary fact that today in the western world, so stricken with obesity, diabetes, heart disease and other illnesses of excess, that many people are malnourished. Malnourishment of our body communicates itself through hunger. If your body hungers for minerals or vitamins that it is not getting, then you will be motivated to eat more food, but if the food that you eat does not provide these nutrients, then you will never be satiated. Malnutrition can cause obesity, and certainly is an underlying cause of diabetes, heart disease, and many other maladies.

I suggest that everyone make an accurate diet menu for a week. Break down the foods that you eat into their raw ingredients. For example; toast with jam for breakfast= wheat, sugar, strawberries, pasta and salad for lunch= wheat, tomatoes, onions, oregano, vegetable oil, parmesan cheese (dairy), lettuce, cucumber, avocado and tomatoes, cookies with coffee for a snack = coffee (stimulant) milk (dairy product) sugar, wheat, eggs? (in cookies maybe) and pizza for supper= wheat, dairy product, tomatoes, red peppers, onions.

Make this list for a week and add up the number of ingredients you think you consume on average every day. This is easier to do when you prepare your own meals as you will be acutely aware of seasoning. The above example, while it may have seemed like a varied diet, with a different tasting food at each meal, there were only a few ingredients, with the majority of the food comprised of wheat, and sugar.

In addition to analyzing the number of ingredients in each day, it is also worth adding up the number of different ingredients in the whole week and then dividing by 7. It is likely that a pattern of a diet heavy in wheat and sugar, dairy, rice, potatoes, corn, and soy will present itself to you.

From here you can look for ways to increase the variety of ingredients that you are exposed to.

Whole foods available to many of us include (by no means an exhaustive list):

Meat: chicken, turkey, quail, pheasant, wood pigeon, duck, goose, lamb or mutton, beef, pork (unless forbidden by your religion) rabbit or hare. In other countries, the following may be found on the menu: alligator, kangaroo, wilder beast, horse, zebra, ostrich, guineapig, donkey, goat, frog legs, elephant, etc.

Insects are also on the menu in many countries from ants to crickets, to grubs, and snails, etc. (remember if it is not dangerous to the body then humans somewhere will probably have eaten them, out of hunger, necessity, and availability)

Animal products: dairy, this includes ghee, butter, yogurt, milk, kefir, cheese (in its many varieties). Although the majority of people associate dairy with cows milk, there are a number of products available made from goats milk, sheeps milk, buffalo milk and others (yak's milk in Mongolia and reindeer milk in Siberia). Eggs: chicken, duck, ostrich, quail, goose, turkey, (nothing endangered please). Honey is considered an animal product.

Fish and seafood: caviar, roe, sardines, cod, salmon, trout, tuna, mackerel, prawns, crabs, lobster, crayfish, mussels, clams, oysters, (dolphin, whale, and seal in some parts of the world). Also included: anchovies, catfish, perch, pollock, scallop, shrimp, sole, squid, tilapia, trout, whitefish, clam, flounder, haddock, herring, mullet

Grains: oats, rice, wheat, corn, spelt, barley, buckwheat, millet, quinoa, amaranth, teff, wild rice. There is an ever-growing popularity for the less well-known grains, and many can be found in health food stores.

Carbohydrate-rich roots, fruits, and tubers: potatoes, swedes, parsnips, manioc root, yam, breadfruit, sago, plantain.

Beans and pulses: lentils, red lentils, black beans, pinto beans, broad beans, butter beans, chickpeas, green peas, green beans, kidney beans.

Nuts: Brazil nuts, cashew, pine, walnuts, almonds, pecans, macadamia, hazelnuts, coconuts, pistachios, sunflower. Seeds: linseeds, sesame, poppy, pumpkin, hemp, caraway, cumin, parsley, carrot, fennel, dill, anise.

Fruits: lemon, lime, orange, pomelo, grapefruit, kumquat, pink grapefruit, mandarin, clementine, plum, nectarine each, damson, greengage, apricot, cherry, raspberry, strawberry, maqui, mortilla, cape gooseberry, cranberry, blueberry, goldenberry, goji berry, gooseberry, blackberry, blackcurrant, redcurrant, elderberry, mulberry, acai (and an almost endless number of berries available in different parts of the world, excellent super-food, filled with antioxidants vitamins and nutrients) apples, pears, quince, banana, mangoes, figs, passion-fruits, dates, lucuma, rhubarb, cherimoya, durian, prickly pear, lychee, rambutan, loganberry, mangosteen, papaya, jackfruit, , kiwi fruit, guanabana, pomegranate, grapes, plum yews, watermelon, cantaloupe melon, many other varieties of melon

Vegetables: carrot, onion, leek, beetroot, courgettes, marrow, peppers, broccoli, cauliflower, lettuce, rocket, tomatoes, aubergines, kale, cabbage, kohlrabi, tatsoi, pak choy, celery, celeriac, pumpkin, squash (many of these vegetables are available in many varieties), spinach, chard, avocado pear (although technically a fruit just like tomatoes and cucumbers), asparagus, artichokes, Jerusalem artichokes.

Mushrooms: button, shitake, diwiñe, oyster, field, portobello, chanterelle, maitake, matsutake, truffles, morel.

Seaweed: dulce, kelp, nori, Irish moss, laver, arame, wakame, cochayuyo, spirulina.

"Sea vegetables have lots and lots of minerals: for example, they all have calcium, iron, phosphorus, potassium, manganese, sodium, zinc, and iodine.... They also include vitamins like A, C, and the Bs......Sea veggies actually bind with radioactive substances in the body and release them. People living near Hiroshima and Nagasaki who ate sea vegetables did much better than those who didn't."[5.]

Sea salt or rock salt *"unrefined salt ...provides not only sodium chloride but also magnesium and many trace minerals. Refined salt is devoid of these nutrients and contains an aluminum compound that prevents the salt from clumping, so that it "pours when it rains."* [2.]

Culinary herbs and spices: sage, rosemary, oregano, thyme, basil, coriander, parsley, bay leaves, chiles, curry, turmeric, cinnamon, cardamom, saffron, pepper, cloves, nutmeg, cacao, ginger, garlic, cumin, graham masala, star anise

Sweeteners; raw cane sugar, maple syrup, agave syrup, rice syrup, honey, stevia, raw coconut palm sugar.

There are a great many other whole foods available throughout the world, try to explore the more traditional fruits, herbs, and spices of the region you find yourself. From the above list, it should be quite easy to find a minimum of 30 ingredients every day. Every little helps, why not make hot cocoa with honey to sweeten and add cinnamon or nutmeg? Bake a variety of seeds into your homemade bread and stir-fry some mixed greens and vegetables with garlic, ginger, turmeric, star anise, and other healthy spices.

Did you know that in addition to adding a pleasant flavor, many spices were originally used and valued for their anti-parasitic and antibacterial properties? Large quantities of seasonings, (including salt and pepper) were originally a source of defense against bacteria and parasites from meats preserved without refrigeration.

Many people suffering from depression are lacking necessary B vitamins and nutrients such as niacin and tryptophan. 16 cashew nuts per day provide the daily recommended dose of niacin which have been shown to combat some cases of depression (very helpful in the postnatal period) and are a much better option than taking pharmaceutical antidepressants.

In the Garden

Oriental and Asian cooking often contain a wide variety of stir-fried vegetables and other ingredients. Much of this cooking style and diet has been directly influenced by the availability of fuel (quick cooking, everything chopped small) and the kitchen garden.

If you grow food in your own garden and are familiar with the "cut and come again" style of harvesting, then it is easy and convenient. It is even preferable to gather a little bit of several kinds of leafy green vegetables and leave the plants to continue growing, and producing for a longer period of time than to uproot the whole plant (for quantity) that will then never produce again.

Gardening, and growing your own food, is one of the most rewarding things that you can do. It does take time and effort as well as patience (very good practice for parenting). Supermarkets and markets overflowing with a wide variety of fruits and vegetables year-round will have you thinking that it is almost effortless to produce large quantities of food. However, industrialized food of this nature is often produced in a vast monoculture with the assistance of large quantities of herbicides, pesticides, artificial fertilizers, and machinery. A very different prospect from a back-garden allotment, or a window box herb and salad bar.

Even a little space can produce a contribution to your diet, especially if you choose to buy organic and heirloom seeds.

Heirloom seeds are natural seeds that have not been hybridized or genetically modified; hybridized seeds often will not germinate past 2 or 3 years. Whereas, natural seeds that have been found in sealed Egyptian tombs and other archaeological sites, have been sown and have actually produced healthy living plants, more than 2000 years after they were stored.

"We save the seeds over winter and plant them again in spring. We are midwives to their gifts." [1.]

Gardening will put you more in touch with the cyclical rhythm of your natural environment, putting much of religious and cultural traditions into context. In addition, it will provide you with a greater appreciation, not only for the food that you, yourself, produce (you might be so proud of them that you don't want to eat them) but also for all the food that you consume, especially that is ethically and sustainably produced.

Researchers from Bristol University and University College London discovered that *Mycobacterium vaccae,* a microorganism in healthy soil activated neurons to produce the brain chemical serotonin, which is a natural antidepressant. Working in the earth can make you happier.

"Apart from having a range of pharmacological actions, serotonin constricts blood vessels, sends messages between cells in the brain and within the central nervous system, regulates secretion of digestive juices, and helps to control the passage of food through the gut...Low levels of serotonin are linked with a number of disorders including aggression,

*anxiety, depression, **obsessive-compulsive disorder** (OCD), bipolar disorder, irritable bowel, and **fibromyalgia**."* [7.]

Gardening with one's children provides an excellent education for them, with principals that provide a practical foundation for maths, chemistry, biology, medicine, economics, agriculture, poetry, nutrition, cooking and many other topics. Gardening, specifically, organic gardening in a Permaculture or biodynamic context, should be considered as an essential part of the school curriculum, providing practical healthy skills.

Many Waldorf schools and Montessori schools incorporate child-friendly gardens, and gardening of perennial fruits, nuts, berries, as well as beautiful flowers that inspire the children. Children who actively participate in the production of a garden often experience a greater appreciation for its beauty and are more inclined to be careful of the other life forms they find there, plants, bird, insects (all interesting topics for science projects).

"The land loves us back. She loves us with beans and tomatoes with roasting ears and blackberries and bird songs. By shower of gifts and a heavy rain of lessons. She provides for us and teaches us to provide for ourselves. That's what good mothers do." [1.]

Even if you are limited for space living in a city, there are ways to learn the art of food production. Many small balconies and window boxes have been converted into productive high yielding allotments, and there are many community gardening projects, where the growing popularity of Permaculture has launched many social projects, including volunteer groups that help people to convert their underused lawns to perennial food forests.

The sooner you learn these skills, the easier it will be for you to pass them on to your children. Setting up a healthy lifestyle now ensures a healthy lifestyle for your future family, and for countless generations.

Tao Diet

The Taoist Diet, originating in China, is also based upon whole foods, This is an omnivorous diet, which includes a great variety of herbs and tonics, which are chosen for their strengthening and health-promoting properties rather than palatability. The diet excludes dairy products in general, however, a wide variety of fruits, vegetable grains and meats are included. Meats are more heavily emphasized than in the traditional macrobiotic diet, with a meat or fish ingredient likely being served up twice a day. Every ingredient has associated properties, and different meats, just as different roots and vegetables are often prescribed to patients visiting a Traditional Chinese Medicine practitioner in order to treat specific ailments or restore the balance of energy within the body.

Taoism is a complete philosophy which addresses every area of life. From the energy in one's body, through acupuncture, massage, diet, exercise and lifestyle to energy in the home (often known as Feng Shui) office buildings, landscapes, etc., as well as systems of divination (I Ching) and philosophies of behavior, conduct, and self-discipline. It is a comprehensive and in-depth philosophy on how to live life well which has been developed over thousands and thousands of years. If you are interested, there is a great deal of published material on the subject available for self-study.

My recommendations are towards an entirely (try the very best you can) whole foods diet. Try to incorporate the greatest variety of fresh, organic or biodynamic ingredients that you can find (although not everyone can afford to buy organic all the time, do so whenever you can, and buy lots of fresh foods from a farmers' market and other ethical sources when you can). Large amounts of fresh, raw fruits, vegetables, nuts, and seeds can be consumed throughout pregnancy and while breastfeeding in unlimited quantities.

If you do include meat or fish in your diet, always look for organic, or better yet, free-range or wild (organic and may be fed pellets made from corn and soy which are not their natural foods), since meats and cultivated fish such as salmon often contain residual antibiotics and other nasties. Fish high in mercury; predatory fish such as shark, tilefish, king mackerel, and tuna, should be avoided or limited. Shellfish, and raw fish, such as in sushi, are not recommended during pregnancy due to the risk of contamination that could pass through the placenta and affect the growing fetus.

Eggs are an excellent supplement. Always pick free-range organic eggs as the nutritional value is higher than eggs from battery production systems. Eggs contain Vitamin A, D, E, K_2 Sulphur, Choline, Folate, Biotin and essential minerals like iron, zinc, and selenium, all vital nutrients for reproduction and the growing fetus. *"Egg whites provide perfect protein and egg yolks contain a powerhouse of nutrients, chief among them being choline, which is critical for the development of the brain...Egg yolks are the richest source of choline, containing about 680 mg per 100 grams, or 115 mg per yolk."*[2.]

Always listen to your body and its cravings (for high-quality whole foods) as they are direct signs as to what you and your baby need. I have met some vegan women struggling to conceive, who were successful after introducing eggs to their diet, although this is, of course, controversial, and depends upon the ethics of the individual. Eggs are rich in choline which has been known to contribute to fertility and to maintaining a healthy pregnancy. If you cannot eat eggs, then consider investigating alternative plant-based sources of choline such as broccoli and quinoa or vegetarian/vegan supplements. Fish eggs, such a roe, and caviar also provide excellent sources of nutrients for mothers but need to be thoroughly cooked. Eggs, nuts, and seeds are always powerhouses of nutrients and particularly useful for ensuring the health and productivity of the reproductive organs.

"...fish eggs are rich in vitamins B_{12}, vitamin K_2, cholesterol, choline, selenium, calcium, magnesium, vitamin A, zinc, iodine, trace minerals and DHA- all necessary for healthy reproduction and the development of the endocrine system. The nervous system and the brain. Caviar is also

extremely rich in vitamin D- containing over 10.000 IU per tablespoon" [2.]

Fruits and vegetables should make up the highest proportion of anyone's diet. Choose a variety of whole grains and legumes to satisfy your energy needs throughout the day. Whole grains contain the entire grain kernel- the bran, germ, and endosperm. Refined grains have been milled, a process that removes the bran and the germ. This is done to give grains a more delicate texture and improve their shelf life, but it also removes dietary fiber and other vital nutrients. Try to mix up the grains that you consume, buying rye bread for toast, making porridge out of buckwheat, and choosing spelt wheat pasta or soba noodles (made from buckwheat flour), finding "exotic" grain milks to poor on your whole grain multi-seed berry muesli, etc.

Wild rice is actually a different species from the brown rice one may be accustomed to cooking with and makes a highly nutritious and flavorful addition to the menu. Wild rice is a traditional staple of the indigenous people of the lake districts of North America. Try to find a brand that is privately owned or where profits benefit indigenous communities since this is a traditional source of income and trading amongst these communities, who have dedicated themselves to sustainable and respectful harvesting method for generations.

The choice to consume dairy products depends very much on the individual (some find that sheep milk and sheep's cheese etc. are kinder to the digestion as an alternative to cow's milk). If you have any sensitivity to dairy products, I suggest you cut them out entirely.

Dairy should also be avoided for anyone struggling to conceive, as dairy can produce an excess of mucus in the body, including cervical mucus, which can detrimentally affect sperm mobility within the vagina.

The macrobiotic diet recommends avoiding dairy products as a general rule. *"Don't get down on yourself if, while reading this, you're thinking, "Holy cow, I don't want to give up dairy! I love dairy!" Don't worry. Every dairy lover feels the same way because you are literally, physically, and hormonally bonded to dairy as you are bonded to your mother."* [5.]

Please get into the habit of checking the ingredients list of everything that you buy. The best foods are those that don't need ingredient labels (fruit and veg), or that only use a few recognizable ingredients. Such as raw vegan chocolate which contains cocoa powder, raw cane sugar (unprocessed) and coconut oil or cocoa butter (both natural oils that are solid at room temperature).

Never consume anything with ingredients that you cannot identify and try to use products with as few ingredients as possible.

Soy

There are many vegan alternatives in health food stores. However, I do not recommend soy products. Soy is one of the most mass-produced ingredients invading every corner of the market, with conventional farming spraying crops with astonishing numbers of herbicides, pesticides, and fertilizers. Even organically produced soy products often leave a wake of destruction deteriorating soils and leading to the desertification of vast tracks of previously high yielding soil.

There have also been links between high soy intake and raised estrogen which has been linked in several studies to PMS, painful periods, polycystic ovarian syndrome, breast and uterine cancers, obesity in men and women and hormonal imbalances. Traditional diets that include soy products such as tofu and tempeh limit intake to a couple of times a week and always used soy that has been fermented in some way to de-nurture (break down) the toxins that are an inherent part of the soybean.

Soy, along with corn, wheat, sugar, and potatoes (starch) can be found in most processed foods and are being consumed at alarmingly high levels. Soy is often the basis of dried foods fed to factory bred cows, chickens and other livestock (rather than grass and fresh varieties of grains), which means that soy is the building block of many other unrelated foodstuffs.

"Soy products should be strictly avoided—they are loaded with phytoestrogens that can cause hormonal imbalances and thyroid problems, and oxalates and enzyme inhibitors that can cause extreme digestive distress. In addition, they contain high levels of phytic acid that can block the uptake of important nutrients like zinc, calcium, iron, and magnesium. Phytoestrogens are strong anti-fertility agents that may prevent you from becoming pregnant; and if you consume soy foods while pregnant, these endocrine disruptor's can cross the placenta and have an adverse effect on the fetus. Even at very low levels, exposure to genistein, the main phytoestrogen in soy, caused behavior changes in rodents, including increased signs of stress, decreased social contact and altered sexual development." [2.]

The Mother's Diet

The mother's diet during pregnancy can affect the gene expression of her child. The exciting field of epigenetics is investigating how our environment can influence our DNA. Since our first environment is our mother womb, the chemical composition of the amniotic fluid that we soak in, blood and oxygen flow, and a variety of other components can influence the way that our genetic blueprint manifests in our physical bodies, effectively turning specific gene sequences on or off.

"It is the mother and the nature of the influence that she contributes to her baby's mental development, as well as the

chemical substances that percolate through her placenta, that mold to a large extent, the future of the child. The maternal mental processes during gestation build within her the structure of an offspring after her own form and function."[8.]

Studies conducted on the children of parents who suffered malnutrition, due to war, concentration camps, anorexia and crash dieting during pregnancy, suggested that their offspring were much more likely to develop diabetes, heart diseases, and eating disorders. The reason behind this is that mother nature, kind as she is, adapts the child to the diet of the mother, as this is the expected diet of the child once it is born. The environment that you live in determines not only the types of foods available but also the calorific quantity available. If someone finds themselves in a period of drought or crop failure where rations are severely limited, then the child grows to be especially efficient regarding digestion. The child is created to survive and endure privation, however, if the child who would survive on less is exposed to more, as in much of the western world, then that child will be even more susceptible to the adverse health effects of overindulgence. Even eating a standard calorie-controlled diet, a child who was built to survive on less, may well put on excess weight.

"modern research has shown us that nutrition, in fact, affects the expression of the genes, and poor nutrition can so adversely affect genetic expression that "defects" persist for several generations. The prediction of healthy babies indeed consists of a partnership between ourselves and the creator; God provides the blueprint, the genetic code, while we the

parents, provide the building materials. Together we can build magnificent body temples to house the soul's future generations, the souls who will ensure that peace and justice reign on the earth."[2.]

Never try to diet during pregnancy, or during breastfeeding, as it will limit the quality of nutrients available to your child. Eat many nutrient-dense foods such as sesame seeds for calcium. Sufficient calcium and a varied diet during pregnancy will help to build bone density in the mother, preparing her for later life and resulting in a lower risk of osteoporosis. However, when a woman does not consume enough calcium and other minerals she is at a higher risk of these nutrients being stripped from her bones, teeth, and nails, etc. to feed and build the growing fetus. Many women have lost all their teeth during pregnancy, and this is one of the reasons that dental care is free for pregnant women in the UK.

Superfoods, such as berries, blueberries, goji berries, maqui berries, and raspberries, have a vast number of antioxidants, vitamins, minerals and other essential nutrients, and you should take the opportunity to indulge in them whenever possible. Spirulina is also an excellent supplement high in protein and iron. Dark leafy greens, especially those of rarer varieties (and therefore fewer generations of manipulation to suit modern farming method that results in fast yielding but less nutrient-dense foods) such as kale, Swiss chard, spinach, rocket, and others are rich sources of folate, vitamin B9, and many other nutrients.

Folate vs. Folic Acid

Foliate is especially necessary during pregnancy for the healthy formation of the fetus, which is why folic acid is often prescribed during pregnancy. Folic acid is the synthetic version of the naturally occurring folate and is utilized differently in the body. Folate is metabolized in the stomach, while folic acid is metabolized in the liver.

Many women with a history of miscarriage or trouble conceiving are advised to take double doses of folic acid or take folic acid while trying to conceive. Although this has been proven effective in some cases, there is a potential downside. Increased folic acid intake during pregnancy has been linked to the development of Tongue tie in babies, which although easily resolved, can lead to complication in breastfeeding and speech development if not spotted early enough. Excess folic acid has also been linked to a suppressing of the body's natural killer cells and therefore, a related increase in cancer, specifically breast and colon cancer and may even raise the risk of developing gestational diabetes. The very best source of natural folate is leafy greens and vegetables. To increase your intake, try making green juices or smoothies and adding spirulina (blue-green algae), kale and nori.

Some people are born with a defective MTHFR gene which means that they have a decreased ability to produce a folate called methyl-folate. If you have this defective gene, you should not take folic acid (since it can increase the risk of miscarriage and other serious complications), but rather seek out folinic acid and methyl-folate. A simple blood test can be ordered to find out if you have this mutation.

Try visiting Oriental and Asian supermarkets where you will be able to find a variety of seaweeds, dried shitake mushrooms, and many vegetables, which will add variety to your home-cooked meals. Chinese takeaway food is not necessarily any more nutritious than other fast foods, as businesses are likely to prioritize profit rather than the quality of ingredients, and high levels of monosodium glutamate are added for flavoring. Monosodium glutamate naturally occurs in dairy products, fermented soy products, and human breast milk, it is umami, and it is addictive, it is designed to be. In nature, an infant's addiction to breast milk encourages the child to nurse frequently which is necessary for optimal growth. However, when this compound is isolated and put into processed foods, it can cause people to be addicted to those foods. People trying to quit dairy food will attest to the overwhelming cravings they initially experience. Monosodium glutamate can be found in almost all processed foods and even in simple kitchen items such as stock cubes. Unfortunate monosodium glutamate is a neuron-stimulator, and some children have experienced adverse effects to overdosing on this compound, including suffering brain damage, strokes, and convulsions. It has also been linked to ADHD.

Seaweed is an excellent source of iodine, which is essential for healthy hormone production and a healthy thyroid. Iodine is often missing from table salt which is one of the reasons why it is necessary to use rock salt or sea salt in your cooking. If you experience edema during pregnancy, swelling around the ankles or elsewhere, then it may be helpful to add iodine to your diet. Remember that your child needs it as much as anything else and will take extra from the store of reserves in your body if you do not provide it through your diet. Women are thought to need up to 16 times more iodine in their diet during pregnancy, which may result in salt cravings. Be sure you are using iodized salt or sea salt, etc. Nori (think sushi rolls) and kelp are commonly found seaweeds especially cochayullo (bull kelp) in Chile.

It is possible to overdose on iodine, which can adversely affect the thyroid. One sheet of nori (sushi wrap) per day provides adequate iodine for the average healthy adult.

Mushrooms and other edible fungi, including "Quorn" are a rich source of vegetarian protein. They should be avoided if there is any intolerance to yeast, or if a yeast or fungal infection, such as candida, is present. They often turn up as ingredients in vegetarian dishes and veggie burgers.

Drink plenty of fluids, natural (preferably fresh rather than pasteurized) fruit and vegetable juices, herbal teas, and pure, clean water (remember that tap water may contain contaminants such as fluoride, chlorine, and other nasties). A variety of water filters are available on the market, so be sure to choose carefully something which can filter out chlorine and fluoride.

Avoid caffeine during pregnancy, and if trying to conceive, caffeine strips many minerals from the body, including calcium, magnesium, zinc, and iron, which has been linked to inhibited growth and pre-term labor. Caffeine, is, however, recommended in small quantities for men trying to conceive as it also stimulates sperm performance. (once you have and your partner have conceived show some solidarity with your pregnant wife/ partner and cut out caffeine). Caffeine is also found in tea, and a similar compound is found in Yerba Mate (a favorite drink in South America and elsewhere), smaller doses are found in green tea and cacao. High levels of caffeine intake have been linked to low birth weight and even miscarriage.

Chocolate feeds our womb. Deep dark cacao makes the womb unfurl. It is felt here. Stick to high-quality, high cacao chocolate where possible.

Also, on the list to avoid, during pregnancy include, unpasteurized fermented products, patè, mold-ripened cheeses such as brie, Camembert Stilton or Danish blue cheeses, it is recommended that you only consume pasteurized dairy products and avoid fish with high levels of mercury (as mentioned previously). Be very careful if you decide to consume maternity vitamins that you do not exceed the dose as some vitamins such as vitamin A can be dangerous to your child's development in large quantities.

It is always preferable to get your nutrients, minerals, and vitamins from whole foods rather than from synthetic supplements and vitamin tablets. *"the earth doesn't produce nutrients in capsule form or as free-floating entities to be jammed into "health-food" products. Nature produces whole foods, and the vitamins and minerals therein are balanced and absorbable when eaten in their original package. When we break a natural organism into bits and pieces, extracting this and that, we create an imbalance in the organism. When we then feed ourselves these extractions for added nutritional oomph, we create imbalances in ourselves.* "[5]

On the list of things to avoid indefinitely, for a healthy family and setting a good example for yourself and your children are No alcohol and No drugs. Even try avoiding prescription drugs and over the counter pharmaceuticals (paracetamol and ibuprofen are not considered safe during pregnancy). No smoking. No exposure to pesticides, herbicides, radiation, or heavy chemicals such as paint fumes of hairdressing products. *"Especially dangerous are cholesterol-lowering drugs, sometimes promoted to women of child-bearing age. These drugs—called statins—are a Class X teratogenic, meaning that they can cause serious birth defects. If you become pregnant while taking a statin, the damage may be done before you even know you have conceived."*[2]

If you are non-vegan and have the good fortune to raise your animals (in addition to cultivating your crops) for the production of meat, eggs, and dairy products, make sure that all of your animals are free-range, grass-fed animals. Try to avoid their exposure to pesticides, herbicides, and antibiotics, so that the quality of the produce that you harvest of is of the very highest quality for yourself and your family.

"deeply rooted in cultures of gratitude, this ancient rule is not just to take only what you need, but to take only that which is given." [1]

Skin Deep

Now that we have identified the products that we consume by mouth it is worth mentioning that 60% of what we put on our skin is absorbed into the body.

Many of the products that we apply to our skin on a daily basis, soaps, shampoos, detergents, lotions creams, suntan lotion, makeup, hair dyes, toothpaste, perfumes, deodorants, and aftershaves have a large number of toxic metals and dangerous chemicals. We should not want these products to absorb into our bodies and negatively affect our health or the health of our unborn children.

Fluoride, found in toothpaste, is especially dangerous and has been linked to lowering intelligence, endocrine system depletion, atrophy of the pituitary gland, bone and (ironically) dental problems, amongst other contraindications. Fluoride is after all the predominant ingredient in rat poison, and Prozac as well as many other antidepressants. Fluoride was first added to a public water supply in Nazi concentration camps during the Holocaust. The effect of fluoride fed to the population was to make them more docile, and less likely of fighting back. Fluoride is banned from being added to the water supply in several countries, including Japan, the Netherlands and other Scandinavian countries. If you wish to avoid fluoride in toothpaste, you can find fluoride-free toothpaste in health-food stores or make your own from a recipe online. You will want to consider removing fluoride toothpaste from your house when little ones come along, as one tube of toothpaste has enough fluoride to kill a small child. This is why a warning is placed on the tube in case a child ingests the toothpaste.

Aluminium used in deodorants has been linked to breast cancer, thankfully, there are natural alternatives available, ranging from bicarbonate of soda to special rock deodorants made from mineral compounds. Synthetic perfumes are often filled with toxins, and many pregnant women, with an increased sensibility of smell, will feel nauseous when exposed to the scent of strong perfumes. This can be a nightmare on crowded transportation systems, where it seems that everyone is wearing a different scent.

Alternative natural perfumes can quickly be prepared from essential oils used in aromatherapy (purchase only pure essential oils, not just aromatherapy or massage oils which are often diluted or synthetic). Each oil, just like each plant, will have associated medicinal properties, just as they have different fragrances. Be careful, as there are some oils that are best to avoid during pregnancy. Essential oils are a concentrated essence of the plant and as good as they smell some of them can be irritating to the skin (such as cinnamon, bergamot or tea-tree oil).

Ni, Daoshing, and Herko, Dana in the book The Tao of fertility, list the following ingredients as those to avoid when purchasing skin care, beauty and cleaning products:

"imidazolidinyl urea, diazolidinyl urea, methyl paraben, propyl paraben, butyl paraben, ethyl paraben, petrolatum, propylene glycol, PVP VA copolymer, stearalkonium chloride, synthetic colors, synthetic fragrances, diethanolamine (DEA), monoethanolamine (MEA), triethanolamine (TEA), dioxane, 2-bromo-2-nitropropane-1. 3-diol (bronopol), benzalkonium chloride, butylated hydroxyanisole (BHA), butylated

hydroxytoluene (BHT). Chloromethylisothiazolinone, and isothiazolinone."[9.]

Many natural products from perfumes to soaps, shampoos and creams can be found which use natural ingredients and fragrances provided by pure essential oils. These are the better alternative. Start clearing out the chemical laden products from your home and replacing them with natural options from your local health food store, online, or you may like to take a course to try to learn to make your own. Baby products such as stretch mark cream, nappy cream, and other products are also available; it is worth checking out sources in advance for a healthy natural start to your baby's hygiene care.

Natural soaps, for example, can be made from fat (either animal fats or vegetable oil, or combinations of both) and lye (either potassium hydroxide for liquid soaps and shampoos or sodium hydroxide for solid soaps and shampoo bars) with other ingredients added for benefits such as scent, color, exfoliation, antibacterial properties etc.

"Think of it this way—your skin is the largest organ of your body, and it literally sucks stuff in. So, when I am buying a skin-care product, I read the label and ask myself if I would be comfortable drinking the ingredients, because slathering them on my body is almost the same thing." [5.]

Conclusion

When you take care of your body and your health, then you are taking care of the health of your children and providing the quality of life that you and your family will share in the future. Positive nutrition is not just for pregnancy; it is not temporary. By adopting positive eating habits now, you make healthy choices the norm for your future children and enable them to start their lives as optimally as possible.

Feed your children love, and nurture them with appreciation. Thank you, and I love you are the greatest foods for their soul. When we love and love fully, we bless everything that we do, everything we say, everyone, we are with and everything we eat.

Love your food, and say Thank you, for all those who contributed to sustaining you here on earth.
Blessings

Bibliography

1. Braiding Sweetgrass, Robin Wall-Kimmerman

2. The Nourishing Traditions Book of Baby & Child Care Morell, Sally Fallon; Morell, Sally Fallon; Cowan, Thomas S.; Cowan, Thomas S.

3. The Bible Diet and Scary News on the Meat YOU Eat! www.beliefnet.com

4. The Crone, women of age wisdom and power by Barbara G. Walker

5. The Hip Chick's Guide to Macrobiotics: A Philosophy for Achieving a Radiant Mind and Fabulous Body by Jessica Porter

6. Gut and Psychology Syndrome (GAPS), By Natasha Campbell-McBride, www.westonprice.org

7. Soil Bacteria Work in Similar Way to Antidepressants Written by Catherine Paddock Ph.D.

8. Childbirth Without Fear: The Principles and Practice of Natural Childbirth by Grantly Dick-Read

9. The Tao of Fertility: A Healing Chinese Medicine Program to Prepare Body, Mind, and Spirit for New Life by Ni Daoshing and Herko, Dana

About the Author

Mrs. Jemmais Keval-Baxter resides in Chile with her family. She is a Natural Childbirth Coach, Doula, Doula Trainer, Writer, and EFT Coach. For more information about her books and workshops, please consult her website at **www.hooponoponodoula.com**.

Did you enjoy this book?
Would you like to read more from
Jemmais Keval-Baxter
The Ho'oponopono Doula™?

Visit: www.hooponoponodoula.com and
sign up for the mailing list to receive
Free resources and information about
workshops, books, services, and events.

Other books in the series include:
A Doula's Guide to Education
A Doula's Guide to The Placenta
A Doula's Guide to Breastfeeding
A Doula's Guide to Menstruation

Also, by Jemmais Keval-Baxter
Ho'oponopono Birth: Meditations on
Ho'oponopono for Pregnancy and
Childbirth

If you liked this book, please leave a
review so that others can find it too.

Printed in the USA
CPSIA information can be obtained
at www.ICGtesting.com
LVHW060243260824
789260LV00007B/394

9 781999 807146